I FEEL

Good

Real Life Testimonies From People Who Used
Food as Medicine

PRESENTED BY
#1 BEST-SELLING AUTHOR DR. BRENDA T. BRADLEY

Dr. Brenda T. Bradley

I FEEL
Good

Real Life Testimonies From People

Who Used Food as Medicine

Presented By:
Dr. Brenda T. Bradley

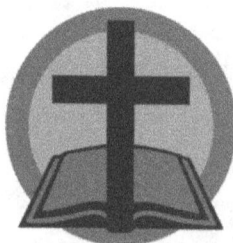

Pearly Gates
Publishing LLC
"Inspiring Christian Authors to BE Authors"

Pearly Gates Publishing, LLC, Houston, Texas

I Feel Good

I Feel Good

Real Life Testimonies From People
Who Used Food as Medicine

ISBN 10: 1-945117-97-4
ISBN 13: 978-1-945117-97-8
Library of Congress Control Number: 2017960534

For information and bulk ordering, contact:
Pearly Gates Publishing, LLC
Angela R. Edwards, CEO
P.O. Box 62287
Houston, TX 77205
BestSeller@PearlyGatesPublishing.com

DEDICATION

This book collaboration is dedicated to all who are firm believers and realize that to achieve anything requires faith, hard work, determination, and a strong belief in oneself.

A *"SPECIAL"* thanks to all the courageous co-authors who dedicated their time to share their personal testimonies in the quest to help others. This is truly an honor to share this platform with each of you.

Many Blessings,

Dr. Brenda T. Bradley

ACKNOWLEDGEMENTS

First and foremost, I give praise and honor to **God** for giving me the ability and strength to stay the course and to listen and obey.

With much gratitude, I must send this special 'Thank You' to my **friends and family** for their ongoing support, encouragement, and love.

Thank you to all the **co-authors** from all walks of life who joined *The 21-Day Vegan Challenge* and are now sharing their personal testimonies with the world. This anthology would not have been possible without each of you. Your decision to boldly step forward to help spread the message will always be appreciated and never forgotten.

There are **many people** around the world who have sent me their testimonies of how *The 21-Day Vegan Challenge* restored their health—and even saved some of their lives. Their testimonies are what continue to inspire me to keep on going!

Dr. Brenda T. Bradley

Last but certainly not least, I can't close without acknowledging my favorite Bible verse:

"I beseech you therefore, brethren, by the mercies of God, that ye present your bodies a living sacrifice, holy, acceptable unto God, which is your reasonable service. And be not conformed to this world; but be ye transformed by the renewing of your mind, that ye may prove what is that good, and acceptable, and perfect will of God."

Romans 12:1-2, KJV

To God be *all* the glory forever!

INTRODUCTION

A NOTE FROM DR. BRENDA T. BRADLEY

Have you ever had a dream sort of like a premonition? At the age of 15, I experienced the worst dream **ever**. In the dream, many people—including family and friends—were sick and dying. No one could explain why.

That dream haunted me for over 34 years. It wasn't until I experienced some devastating moments in my life when I realized the dream was a reality.

When I graduated from high school, I decided to aim high by joining the United States Air Force. I enjoyed being in the military and the opportunities serving provided. One of the number one requirements of the military was to stay physically-fit. Being the "tomboy" that I am, that was not a problem for me.

Many years after leaving the military, I found myself on a battlefield unrelated to the Air Force. Like others, I had fallen victim to obesity. Prior to gaining weight, I was very comfortable in my size 10; but over the course of time, I painfully witnessed my size increase from 10 to

12…14…16…18. I no longer weighed 160 pounds. As if weighing in at 236 pounds wasn't bad enough, I struggled with high blood pressure, high cholesterol, and was pre-diabetic. The dream of my sick and dying family and friends began to slowly emerge as my reality, but I wasn't going down without a fight.

Instead of going to the gym two to three days a week, I continuously increased my visits to the point where I was going four to five days a week — *twice a day*. I went in the morning before work and in the evening after work. I wasn't concerned about the food I was eating because I knew it was all 'healthy'. A sample dinner menu consisted of: red beans and rice, cornbread, fried chicken, a slice of pie with ice cream, and homemade sweet tea. I prepared my own food and very seldom ate out.

Despite my own efforts to lose the weight and keep it off, I secretly joined multiple weight-loss centers and tried many products. **Still, I couldn't get the weight off and keep it off!**

One day, I decided to do something **totally** out of the norm. During Lent (the 40-day religious observance of fasting and repentance during the Spring), my goal was to give up meat, including fish, eggs, milk, and cheese — for only 40 days! After 40 days, I had lost 33 pounds! To celebrate my victory, I treated myself to one of those meals I was used to eating. As soon as I took my first bite of fish, I immediately became sick to my stomach. Not fully understanding what that reaction was all about, the following week, I tried again…and immediately became sick to my stomach. I mentioned this to my brother, Jarvis, and he told me that my body had given up meat and that I was turning into *"one of those Vegan people"*.

Feeling good about the weight loss but confused about what to do prompted me to do my own research on food. What I learned was that food could be a weapon **for** *or* **against** my body.

So, me: ***A Vegan?*** You mean to tell me that for the rest of my life, I will have to eat fruits, vegetables, nuts, grains, and legumes? **Seriously: Who does that?** Forty days was long enough, *BUT* the weight was coming off, staying off, and my health issues were improving. I decided to check out *"those Vegan people"*. I needed to know who they were, where they lived, and where in the heck they were getting their protein from!

One day, while attending a Vegan cooking class, the host announced that she was going to show us how to prepare and cook cornbread, sweet potato fries, greens, and mac-n-cheese. I

immediately raised my hand because I knew how to make mac-n-cheese — and there was *nothing* "Vegan" about it.

"Excuse me. Did you say we are going to make mac-n-cheese and, if so, is this a Vegan cooking class?" I inquired. Her response was **"Yes!"** to both questions. As I sat there, I was amazed to learn that I would still be able to eat some of the foods I loved. When I left that class, I had learned a whole new way of preparing and cooking food. From that day forward, I continued to study and research the power of food.

The Standard American Diet (SAD) is the typical diet of the majority of Americans: high in meat, dairy, fat, and sugar. This "diet" is known to cause high blood pressure, high cholesterol, and diabetes. For African-Americans, this "diet" is the contributing cause for many preventable diet-related illnesses and is plaguing many communities while claiming lives at an alarming rate. The Vegan diet, on the other hand, consists solely of plant-based foods and is totally devoid of all animals and animal by-products — eggs, milk, and cheese. Vegan diets have been associated with **lower** blood pressure, **no form** of diabetes, and **lower** cholesterol levels — just to name a few.

It has been over five years since I changed my diet. I have lost the weight and kept it off. I am not pre-diabetic. I no longer suffer with high blood pressure nor high cholesterol. I truly **FEEL GOOD!**

Excessive weight and illnesses are crippling our society. My problem wasn't underperforming nor overperforming at the gym; it was the **food** I was eating that contributed to my health issues. The dream I had when I was only 15 years old is, in fact, today's reality for countless individuals. Far too many people are sick and dying. Through my work and passion for healthy eating, I answered the call to become a Certified Health Coach. My goal is to inspire, encourage, and motivate others to lead the charge for healthy eating and exercise.

In 2016, I developed a program called *The 21-Day Vegan Challenge*. The program is designed for **anyone** desiring to make a lifestyle change or to explore the healthy benefits of a Vegan diet. Client after client has responded to the Challenge with positive results, both inside and out. I believe that a plant-based diet not only contributes to weight loss, but also improved attitudes as people feel much better about themselves.

I Feel Good is an anthology compiled with the personal testimony of each author. The intent here is to encourage and inspire the people around them who read this book in an effort to raise awareness and become resilient in their own lives. I ask that you simply keep an open mind to the possibility that, when it comes to your health, you should make it a top priority — even if you must take the road less-traveled.

Prior to their testimonies, each author joined *The 21-Day Vegan Challenge*. On the pages that follow, you will find personal stories, many of which are being shared publicly for the first time. Each individual allowed food to become their medicine; not their poison — and we all **FEEL GOOD!**

After reading their stories, I encourage you to take a few minutes to reach out to each of them. If you know someone who is struggling with a similar situation related to any of these testimonies or if you would like to make a gift of books to any specific organization that encourages healthy lifestyles, please reach out to me or the authors.

~ *Dr. Brenda T. Bradley* ~

Meet Dr. Brenda T. Bradley

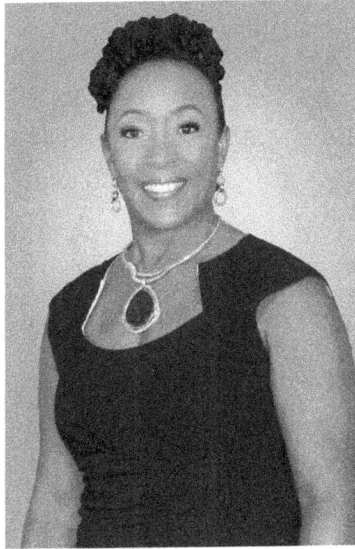

Brenda T. Bradley, PhD, is an engaging and compassionate Certified Integrative Nutrition Health Coach. Through her work and passion for healthy eating and living, she decided to answer the call to become a Certified Health Coach. Determined to break free from the Standard American Diet (SAD)—which is known to do more harm than good—she set out on her journey to research food, diseases, and fitness. Her drive and determination led her to become more involved in health and fitness.

After struggling with her own health goals and learning about the body and what it needs to perform optimally, Dr. Bradley made the switch to a plant-based diet. She credits this diet for helping her to not only lose weight, but it has also improved her overall quality of life. In 2016, she developed a new program, *The 21-Day Vegan Challenge,* and has recommended that clients and those struggling with weight or health issues give it a try. The 21-Day Vegan Challenge is a vegan-only good challenge that stresses the healing power of food and how its proper use can restore the body to a natural, healthy state. Dr. Bradley's goal is to inspire others to lead the charge for healthy eating and exercise. She leads workshops on nutrition and offers individual health coaching, is an inspirational Speaker, and a Best-Selling Author.

Connect with Dr. Brenda T. Bradley:

Website: www.drbtbradley.com

Facebook: www.facebook.com/drbrenda.bradley.121

Twitter: www.twitter.com/drbrendabradley

Instagram: www.instagram.com/docbrad67

TABLE OF CONTENTS

Dr. Brenda T. Bradley

Not My Chicken and Gummi Bears, Too!
By Lenister Brown

L ife has been good to me; great career, family, and friends. I served in the United States Air Force for over 20 years. Exercise was a regular part of my life — coupled with eating "on the go", grabbing 'this' and 'that' without concern of the contents. Then, that chapter of my life closed: less exercise and a more sedentary lifestyle set in. One habit I didn't break was not worrying about what I was eating.

If you talk to many military retirees, they will tell you about the *'Retiree 20'*. That's the 20 pounds you put on in the first few months of retirement. I put on those 20 **plus** five more and moved myself from a comfortable 205 active-duty weight to a 230-pound not-so-happy-or-healthy 44-year-old man. I began taking pre-hypertension medication and then, after my February 2017 visit to the doctor, the doctor said, *"Mr. Brown, you are pre-diabetic"*. Hearing those words and talking to my best friend about eating better and taking better care of myself — not just for me, but also my family — I knew I had to do **something**. That *'something'* was reaching out to Dr. Bradley.

After sitting with my doctor and having her explain some of the medical options I could take (primarily, getting on the medication merry-go-round), I knew that was not for me. I have a young son who needs me more than ever as he starts his journey in life. So, I knew I had to make a change. I always said to my friends, *"I am **NOT** becoming a Vegan, plant-based, or whatever you leaf-lovers want to call yourselves. I'm not giving up my chicken! I had given up beef and pork over 20 years ago. Isn't that enough?"* Obviously, it wasn't. Along with a healthy love for gummi bears, I was killing myself slowly but surely. I needed to reverse the downward spiral I had begun.

Working out in the gym three to four days a week and seeing no progress, I heard all the time: *"You have to change your diet if you want to see progress."* I figured I would outrun these "PRE" diseases that were chasing me down. After a fun weekend in Las Vegas on Super Bowl weekend, I said to myself, *"I **have** to make a change. The change has to be a drastic, lifesaving type of change"*.

The change was going to begin with *The 21-Day Vegan Challenge*.

Enter in Day 1 of 21. Mind you: I don't cook, don't do much grocery shopping, and **never** bring my lunch to work (let alone breakfast). The day before, I went out grocery shopping to gather the things I would need to survive the next 21 days. I packed my breakfast that morning: oatmeal and fruits. I knew I would be fine until lunch. Then came my first **real** challenge;

walking past the chicken bar at my local grocery to get to the salad bar. *Why are the healthy foods always hidden behind the unhealthy items?* There are large displays of chips, cookies, and sodas as **soon** as you walk into the grocery store. Fruits and vegetables are always in the back corner...right next to the bakery. I guess the grocery store must be working hand-in-hand with the pharmacy industry to keep poisoning our bodies. Moving on, I fought past those delicious-looking fried chicken wings (glazed with barbecue sauce) to arrive at the salad bar. There I stood. I grabbed the container and loaded it with spinach, broccoli, cucumber, peppers (green, red, yellow, and orange), edamame, and chick peas. I have never in my life put oil and vinegar on a salad with all the other options staring me in the face and screaming, *"Pick **ME**! Pick **ME**!"* I put a little oil and vinegar on my salad, headed for the register, and checked out. I headed back to the office to eat my salad and (in my mind) starve to death. However, to my surprise, with my sticking to the routine and eating as directed by the plan, I wasn't hungry. I had my *cravings*, but I wasn't **hungry**.

I don't have Facebook, so I didn't have the support of the group to carry me through the next 21 days. Dr. Bradley was that supportive person I needed in my corner who wanted to see me succeed. She called me to see how my first day went.

I have will-power, so I wasn't too concerned about whether I would survive the first week. I survived the first week: no cheating, no falling off the wagon, no jumping off the program. I had seven days in my rearview mirror and was receiving my support calls and texts from Dr. Bradley. I told myself after the first week, *"This isn't too bad!"*

Week two started and I was **ready**! Then came my gummi bear cravings. They are my comfort food, my fun food, my quick snack, and my go-to when I don't want anything healthy. There they were...sitting on the counter: Gourmet Gummies (the good ones). I wouldn't throw them away, just in case I decided this whole 'Vegan thing' wasn't for me. You **know** I'm not giving up my leather belts, shoes, or car seats, so let's just say "plant-based diet". I continued to push through, no longer being tormented by the chicken wings at the grocery store or the gummi bears on my counter at home. Now, mind you: I still had a 9-year-old son with an activity every day. He had to eat, and asking him to make these sacrifices as I did was a bit much (he didn't push back *too* hard when I took away the fast foods from him for 21 days).

We all go through life making changes here and there. Some decisions are small and have no effect on anyone but you; others are large. My decision to accept a plant-based lifestyle was a large decision that would bring positive change to my life by improving my overall health and outlook while educating not only myself, but others around me. I shared my challenges with my family, friends, and coworkers. The person this change would affect the most (besides me) is my wife. She prepares our meals and does the grocery shopping. Now, she must adjust her meals to accommodate me as well as her and our son, Logan. Going through this process was good for all of us.

On day 17 of the Challenge, I decided I would change my life forever. I was going to continue the plant-based lifestyle. It was during those first 17 days that I found many places to eat and how to eat at places I had been to many times before.

If you want to make a change, you just have to take that first step. I made that first step and never looked back. I have one regret: not taking this step **sooner**. *Why did I have to wait until my doctor told me I needed to make some changes?* What **type** of changes was extremely vague, but I knew I needed to make them.

I started this journey at 230 pounds. I thought I was somewhat healthy. Now, I am 195 pounds and feel really good about myself and how I feel. Now, there are a few changes I had to make that must be noted here. I exchanged tips with my best friend all the time. *Why didn't he let me know my entire wardrobe would need to be replaced?* I have purchased more pants, shirts, and belts to replace all the clothes that no longer fit. I'm not complaining because I shouldn't have let myself get in a situation of even having to wear those larger sizes.

Today, I can say I am stronger and have more energy than I have had in an extremely long time. I get up in the morning, never feel tired, workout, and have plenty of energy. There was a false concern in my mind that I need lots of protein to lift weights and continue my workout routine. I have not missed a beat in the gym. If anything, I look better and feel better before **and** after my workouts. After each meal, I never feel stuffed and I know that the foods I am eating are good not only for my body, but my mind as well. I have added natural juices as well.

For those thinking about taking this journey…buy extra toilet paper! ☺

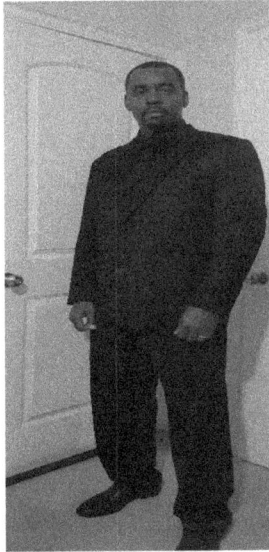

Lenister Brown is a Contract Procurement Specialist, supporting the Air National Guard. He is a Retired Air Force Veteran, after serving for 21 years. During his tenure, he served in the Gulf War, Global War on Terrorism, and in Afghanistan. He holds a Bachelor's Degree in Homeland Security and a Master's in Business Administration with a Concentration on Supply Chain Management. He graduated Summa Cum Laude.

Lenister lives in Brandywine, Maryland.

Contact Lenister Brown

Email: LenisterBrown@yahoo.com

THIS PAGE INTENTIONALLY LEFT BLANK

Get Outta My Way, "Dunlap"!
By Denise Thrash

In life, many events influence the way we act or the decisions we ultimately make. Basically, you can go through certain events in life that have such an impact, they can or will change your whole life's course.

For me, as a child, my mother was often sick and taking several kinds of pills a day. Our bathroom medicine cabinet did not have lotions, perfumes, or other toiletries; it was filled with all kinds of prescription medications. So, as a child, that appeared to be an expected "look" for **ALL** medicine cabinets. As I got older, I knew that any medicine cabinet filled with all kinds of prescription medications was not to be expected nor healthy. As an adult, I did not want *MY* bathroom medicine cabinet to be filled with pills—as I witnessed growing up.

I was born in the deep South: Mobile, Alabama. My siblings are: Ann (the oldest); I'm Denise (the middle child); and my younger brother is Bill. We also have a younger sister named Christina, who is 13 years younger than me. We had some of the best prepared meals cooked by one of the best southern cooks; our mother, Emma. I kid you not: Emma could **COOK**!

We **always** had three meals every day. Breakfast consisted of grits, eggs, bacon or sausage or fried Spam, buttered biscuits made from scratch, and juice. Cold cereal was never an option since we rarely had milk, other than the canned pet milk my mother used for baking and for making her famous macaroni and cheese and cornbread. Lunch consisted of our previous night's dinner or a sandwich—not just cold meat sandwiches, either. Any leftover chicken or turkey would be removed from the bone, cut and seasoned (mixed with bell peppers, onions, carrots, pickled relish, and mayo). In addition, we had a seasonal fruit, raisins, or a slice of homemade pie or cake. For dinner, we always had white rice, fresh seasonal vegetables or dry beans, a meat (i.e. chicken, beef, or pork), and some kind of bread made from scratch. Every Friday, fish was on the menu. Needless to say: The stove was always burning in our house!

Being raised with southern values and roots, we ate from the trees and fields that our parents cultivated and grew. There were not places for "people of color" to dine, so our meals were cooked and consumed at home. After my mother divorced my father, she decided to move my siblings and me to Washington, DC so that she could attend college. Besides, the new city provided many opportunities for my mother, and she wanted the best opportunities for her children. Best of all, my mother had the help of several family members already residing in Washington, DC; ones ready to assist her with getting settled in.

When we moved from Alabama, we rode on a Greyhound bus from Mobile to Washington, DC late at night. That was a **very** long ride. I recall waking up to daylight…still on the bus. We were in a place called Eastover that had clothing stores, a bowling alley, and fast food restaurants located in Oxon Hill, Maryland. We had never seen anything like that in Alabama. My mother said, *"Look at that place!"* What she pointed out was a placed called 'Jack in the Box' — a fast food chain that sold burgers, fries, and sodas (none of which we had *ever* eaten before). My mother told us that if we were good, she would take us there one day. We were so excited at the chance to go because it looked like a fun place for kids to eat!

The new life for my mother consisted of raising three children alone, attending college, and working; however, that did not stop her from making three hot meals a day for her family. When she received her paycheck every other week, she would pack all of us up in her car to go grocery shopping. Before going home, she would stop for dinner at Ponderosa Steakhouse, Red Barn, or Hot Shoppe. Remember: The options were plenty in Washington, DC. The fast food was a treat, easy for my mother, and the food was great!

That was the beginning of a lifestyle-change for our family...

As a single parent, my mother worked hard, managed her college studies, cared for her three children, and participated in countless church activities — from bible study, prayer night, rehearsals, singing in various choirs and groups, to ushering her children from one church to another (and it wasn't always locally). Oftentimes, dinners would consist of whatever the church we visited provided.

Let me take you back to a late Spring day...

The 3:00 p.m. dismissal bell rang at Draper Elementary School. It was total chaos with kids trying to leave the building to head home. My siblings and I had to wait for one another so that we could walk home together, as did all the kids with siblings. For us, it was a 20-minute walk from school to home. On this day, I recall the smell of dinner being prepared, long before reaching our apartment building. The smell was coming directly from our open kitchen window! Just as I opened the front door to the building, I knew what was being prepared. The aroma in the hallway that was wafting through the air was very familiar. The smell made me so hungry! I couldn't wait for the meal to be served (that night, it was fried chicken). I would always try to guess what was for dinner before coming into the apartment by the smell. If it was chicken, I would say, *"Ma, are you cooking chicken?"* She would answer, *"Yes!"* Most of the time, I was correct in guessing, and my mother would say, *"You have a good nose for food"*. She knew my favorite food was fried chicken and fried pork chops smothered in brown gravy with butter beans, rice, and cornbread. I have always belonged to the 'Clean Plate Club'. I can say my mother never cooked a bad meal. We never got fat, either. That's the truth. However, the home-cooked meals prepared by my mother became less frequent due to her increased illness.

Over the last several years, my life has been shaken up by family death, illness, and personal circumstances. I was stressed. I knew that a change had to happen. My mother passed away due to complications from diabetes on the day before Thanksgiving in 2008. I tried tirelessly to get her to change her eating habits to reverse the diabetes, but she simply wouldn't. The diabetes skipped my older sister and me, but is now a part of life for my brother, my youngest sister, and my daughter. This frightens me so much. I do not want diabetes to claim another family member's life. For my daughter, if a lifestyle-change does not happen, the diagnosis could claim her life, leaving me to raise her two young children.

As a Licensed Realtor, I meet people from different walks of life. In June 2013, I met the beautiful Dr. Brenda Bradley. I was her realtor and, as life would have it, I did not know the impactful role she would have on my life and that of my daughter. Dr. Bradley did not reveal to me that she was a Health Coach until a year later. She kept her gift of living a plant-based lifestyle in silence; however, I had also become her friend on Facebook. One day, I read a post on Dr. Bradley's page about her Vegan journey. She posted a discussion about her *21-day Vegan Challenge*. I inquired: *"What is The 21-Day Vegan Challenge and why a Vegan lifestyle?"* She shared with me a traumatic experience she had with her weight and all the diet plans she tried with only temporary results. **Wow!** What a tearful story! After sharing her story, she said to me, *"Denise, you could stand to lose some weight and lose that belly of yours. It's not healthy."* She said that in a way that **only** a friend could say. I immediately said, *"I do not need to lose weight, but I could stand to lose the 'Dunlap Belly'!"* We laughed and laughed!

We continued to discuss the benefits of *The 21-Day Vegan Challenge*. I was thinking more about my daughter as we talked. The Challenge really got my attention. For my daughter, I did not want some yo-yo diet. I inquired about taking Dr. Bradley's Challenge more and more. I was looking for a healthy option void of pills for both my daughter and me. I wanted to make

[14]

sure we could do the Challenge together **AND** be successful. My beautiful daughter has had a few health challenges in her life, but losing weight was by far her biggest challenge. She tried prescription medication. I asked her to stop taking the pills and watch what she ate. I did not want her dependent on prescriptions to control her weight, especially after witnessing what pills did to my mother over the years.

After *The 21-Day Vegan Challenge*, I had lost a total of 16 pounds. The 'Dunlap Belly' was no more—and my daughter lost 22 pounds and counting. My daughter's doctor wanted to know what it is that she's doing differently. She may be able to come off the pills that control her diabetes soon! We now have the right tools to maintain and control the weight and health issues.

When we left Alabama for Washington, DC, did we leave some valuable lessons behind? Perhaps we did. Our course in life has now changed for the better by eating wholesome again.

I want to thank Dr. Bradley and pray she continues to educate people about a plant-based lifestyle and its benefits for one's health and life. She is really helping to save lives—**no prescriptions needed!**

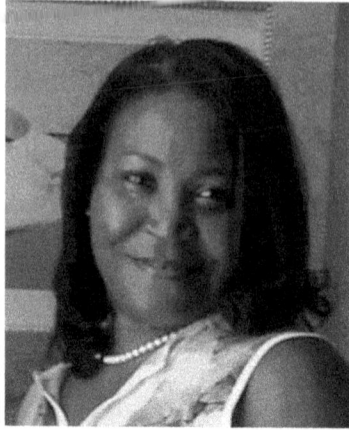

Denise Thrash is a Licensed Realtor in Maryland and the District of Columbia (D.C.). Due to her hectic work schedule, she admits to paying little attention to her nutritional balance. After gaining a few extra unwanted pounds, having her mother pass away from complications associated with diabetes, and learning of her daughter's diabetes diagnosis, Denise made a lifestyle change. Through support from Dr. Brenda Bradley's *The 21-Day Vegan Challenge*, she lost the weight and is happy to report that her daughter's health has taken a turn for the better as well.

Denise states: *"**The 21-Day Vegan Challenge** has broken an unhealthy family cycle, educated her on how to replace bad food for healthier options (without meat), and I am now setting a good example for my family to live healthier lives."*

Contact Denise Thrash

Email: EDeniseThrash@gmail.com

Sacred Soul...Scripted Blessings...Cured by Nature
By Dr. Tiffany Taft

I walk by faith and not by sight. I know there's more, although the path is not always clear. Physically and emotionally disconnected at times, I desired to live a fuller and meaningful life on purpose. I believe in the healing power of God and prayer, and am forever grateful for the grace and mercy He gives me every day with the opportunity to "get it right". I am a living testimony that I do not look like what I've been through. Years of life lessons have born an amazing transformation of love and a purpose-driven life to share my gift with the community. I am honored and humbly hold the sacred space for others to live, realize their own truths, and be unashamed to be their authentic selves.

When I look back at my journey and each significant milestone, I can now tell my 12-year-old self, *"It was just the beginning; keep living!"* I can now tell my 21-year-old self, *"You will survive...and you are!"* I can tell my 30-year-old self, *"You're stronger than you know; you're a warrior!"* And I can tell my 40+-something self, ***"I am loving the woman you're becoming. You are loved!"***

I have a background and have been trained in the ways of Western Medicine from a clinical perspective. I have loved

[17]

healthcare since I was six years old. I love all things 'health and wellness'. I have evolved to embrace and seek out alternatives from ancient wisdoms of Eastern Medicine through yoga, massage, mindfulness, and meditation—along with a host of other holistic therapies that have served me well over the years. While there is an absolute time and place for pills, surgery, and other Western medicinal approaches, I am a strong believer and advocate of choice and prevention that addresses the core of *DIS-EASE* in the body. There is a science to our being. We have been perfectly designed. Every breath, movement, and space of our being has purpose.

As a part of my journey, I knew I had to part from my traditional southern eating and cooking goodness. There is a *REAL* relationship there (😊), but that way of eating is no longer good for me—at least not on a regular basis. I found that I was strong on the outside, but weak on the inside. I am still working on my journey, as it is a daily walk for me; but I can say I am now stronger inside and out because of deliberate action and change to my wellness.

Have you ever just been sick and tired of being **SICK** *and* **TIRED**? How many times did you promise yourself that **TODAY** is the day you commit, do better, and make that change? Did you get to make that decision on your own, or were you like me and your body finally said, **"Enough!"**, and sat you down? It failed you.

That day came for me on *two* separate occasions: once in 2014 and again in 2016. Both times, the symptoms presented exactly the same and the core circumstances were also the same. I was in graduate school working on my PhD full-time, working full time, traveling, doing community service, participating in church activities, and a host of a **LOT** of busyness.

There are things I have learned over the years and through my journey: the power of prayer, the power in saying *"NO"* and being okay with that, and the need for balance, rest, and wholeness. You see, I kept saying, *"There has to be a better way to live – and **LIVE WELL!**"*

My symptoms presented in the physical as stress, body aches, inflammation, and total body pain. I was hurting all the time. It hurt so bad, I didn't want to be touched. I didn't want anything to touch me (clothes, bedsheets, etc.). My body literally felt like it was on fire and like my skin was crawling. I felt like a poorly-aging senior in my 40+-year-old body. If someone could have stuck a straight pin in me, I feel like they could have popped me like a balloon. That's just how tight my skin felt on my frame. If I had to put a modern-day unofficial diagnosis to it. I would call it Fibromyalgia or Lupus. I was never told that it was, but when I found enough strength to begin my healing and was tired of being sick and tired, I decided to do it completely naturally and organic. I said to myself, *"It has to be my food. This food is killing me!"* I was also a statistic, as I suffered with carrying two large cervical fibroids (like many women) for five years that were the size of a four-month pregnancy. I tried all of the Western medicine ways to heal and get rid of them without success. Once again, my body failed me, and I was the walking dead. The foods I ate fed the life of those fibroids while taking life (oxygen and iron) from me.

Honestly, the struggle for me does not come in eating clean, but rather from opportunities to **not** eat that way. I mean, eating out, grocery shopping, cooking…all of it had to change for me. I needed foods that would organically nurture, heal, and sustain me. So, every week, I removed items from my diet that I thought might be the culprit for the body pain and those fibroids; breads, refined sugars, coffee, sweeteners, and more. My biggest relief came when I removed meat—specifically chicken and beef—from my diet. Almost immediately (within five days), I could feel my body again—and it didn't hurt! I was sleeping better, my stress level dropped dramatically, I could move and exercise more, and I even began to drop the toxic weight. My body began to support me with new life when I stopped making it work overtime to keep up with my bad habits.

I thought to myself, *"It was my food!"*

Years of "good eating" and a real relationship with my southern food had turned out to not be the answer for the way I needed to spend the second half of my life. Armed with this new information and feeling better in my body, I began to study and read more in search of what might be a more permanent change I needed to make. As part of this transition and journey, I joined a *21-Day Vegan Challenge*. That was the best decision I could have made for me. Yes, it was a drastic leap to the extreme; but it was a necessary one because I wanted to **live** again. Of course, I checked in with my doctors, but I knew I didn't want their drugs and that it was my food and lifestyle that needed to change. I come from a family like many with "hereditary issues" and "poor diet decisions" that affect one's health, but my story was not like theirs. I somehow managed to escape their common ailments of diabetes, high blood pressure, cholesterol issues, cancers, and more; yet still, something pained me. It turned out I needed to be more plant-based and eat clean.

Since taking the Challenge in 2016 and again earlier in 2017, I can definitely say it works and was not just a coincidence. In the spirit of transparency, I will say that I am about 90% Vegan — meaning I definitely seek those options first in every meal, snack, and opportunity to nourish myself. I am working on being clearer about ingredients, how to prepare the foods, and the trappings of eating out (especially when traveling). By far, this is my greatest challenge. I think I just need my own personal Vegan chef (😊). I am happy I made the decision to eat more ethically and am determined to find the vegan goodness for some of my traditional southern favorite dishes.

Finally, in addition to my diet, I have also taken a closer look at the products I use on my skin and around my home. While the foods I ingested were an issue for my inside, so, too, were the products I used on the outside. I have begun to switch them as well. I believe that we are a physical being having a soulful experience. I know God has provided **EVERYTHING** we need to *naturally* sustain our lives. Yes, He created animals, but He also said, "...*the leaves of the tree were for the healing of the nations*" (Revelation 22:2, KJV).

I hope that my story in some way resonates with you and encourages you to examine and make any change you see fit to eat, live, move, and embrace your whole being. There is no one-size-fits-all, but there is science that proves prevention, clean eating, and conscious living is better. I encourage you to make the choice **today** to live better, be fully present in every moment, and to eat, drink, and be thankful for every new meal you get to eat **WELL**.

I thank you for reading my story, and I support you in your desire to make a change for you. I **AM** a sacred soul of transformation that will continue to empower people to align with their authentic self. I can write this story because I live this story each and every day.

I AM WELL!
I FEEL GOOD!

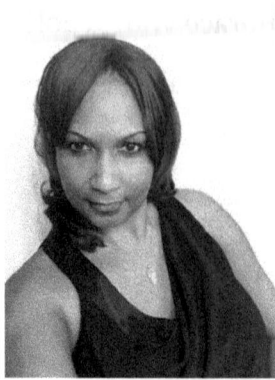

Dr. Tiffany Taft is a Certified Yoga Instructor, Licensed Massage Therapist, and Certified Holistic Health Coach focused on the integration of Eastern and Western medicine approaches to healing for the mind, body, and spirit through Science. Her mission is to be a sacred soul of transformation that will empower people to align with their authentic selves. She has served in the Health and Wellness industry for over 15 years through clinical practice and therapeutic services with private and corporate clients nationwide. Her primary interest is assisting others in achieving their personal and professional goals through self-awareness and mindful connection. She remains an advocate for those who desire to live on purpose.

Dr. Taft provides services (private coaching, yoga and massage services, classes, workshops, etc.) to a variety of clients with a focus on the professional athlete, populations that suffer from chronic pain and rehabilitation issues, and the novice who desires to live better.

Contact Dr. Tiffany Taft

Phone: (703) 677-0339

Email: SacredSoulWellness@gmail.com

Facebook: www.facebook.com/dryogitt

Instagram: @dryogitt and @sacredsoulwellness

In love and light...Namaste!

THIS PAGE INTENTIONALLY LEFT BLANK

Always a Work in Progress
By Ruth Tolbert

This is my 21-Day Challenge testimony. My testimony began back in the 1990s when I was introduced to eating a healthy diet as a young person. All my life, I struggled with endometriosis and infertility issues. I suffered with bad menstrual cycles and had difficulty getting pregnant after being married for seven years. During this time, I learned that stripping my diet of dairy, coffee, and meats would better my health.

The Vegan approach that I took changed my health and I lost weight. Several months later, I conceived my first child. Two years later, I delivered my second child. I naturally-delivered a son **and** a daughter—two healthy babies!

Years later, as life went on and I was enjoying God's gifts of my children, I got 'lost' in raising a family. I became caught up with taking the kids to fast food places where we ate all the wrong foods. Unfortunately, this lifestyle went on for years.

When my daughter was nine years old, my husband took both children to the pediatrician for their annual physical. My husband asked the physicians to do a urine test for both children. My husband had a ketoacidosis event in his 40s which led to the revelation that there was a family history of diabetes to address. Both of our children were pre-disposed to becoming diabetics. The indication of the urine test was that our daughter, Tara, was positive for diabetes. A blood test confirmed the results.

Three years later, we learned that Tara had chronic kidney disease. Everything about her diet, insulin intake, and health needed to be addressed. The doctors told us that by the time Tara was a young lady, she may need a kidney transplant. Everything I thought I knew suddenly became unclear. I didn't know what to do nor how to change my family's food options and choices. Diet plans and all the controversy about processed foods were challenges that we faced as a family.

By age 18, Tara's kidneys were functioning at about 50%. They had deteriorated rapidly. My daughter's health was in jeopardy. I had to do something to change our lives. I felt like we were killing ourselves with food. I started looking on the internet for alternative foods, all the while feeling overwhelmed with all of the information available. The diabetes diet plan was largely about portion-control and consisted of meats, cheese, and carbs.

I felt like I did not know what to do or even where to begin. As years went on, I developed health issues as well; I was diagnosed with high blood pressure, diabetes, and was told that I had bladder cancer. I still had not changed my lifestyle, but that last diagnosis was the straw that broke the camel's back. I had to have my gall bladder removed because everything I ate made me sick. A year after my surgery, I developed a tumor from the removal of the gall bladder (that is quite common).

By this time, my bad eating habits were not yet in control. No matter what I ate, I kept getting sick. My second home was the bathroom. I avoided eating out with friends because of the embarrassing price of excusing myself to go to the ladies' room (I would be in the bathroom for quite a while and I would always feel drained after a bathroom 'episode'). You see, I never knew what would trigger my stomach to go crazy!

It seemed like everyone around me was happy, but I was not happy with me. I was so sad and felt like a failure. I needed help but knew of no one who could help me. I was lost and thought life was being unkind to me. I thought I would **never** find a solution.

My doctor sent me to a Nutritionist, but her recommendations were the same: eat meats in moderation, cheeses, and vegetables. My stomach being upset was still not addressed. Meanwhile, friends and family members seemed to be living a healthier lifestyle than what I was living.

My sister was one of those people who found a better way of eating. I was happy for her. One night after dinner, I got sick and spent most of my time in the bathroom. **I had had enough!** I called my sister to ask her what she had done to lose weight and to look and feel healthy. My sister, Joy, shared with me that she had stopped eating meats and was in the process of eliminating other foods from her diet. I told her, *"I need you to teach me"*. Now, mind you: I had stripped my diet before to get pregnant. I had even shared my information with other women about how to get pregnant by eating better and taking herbs. I explained to my sister that I was desperate. She talked about Dr. Brenda Bradley and her *21-Day Vegan Challenge* and lifestyle program. She explained to me how Dr. Bradley was changing people's lives, just as she helped Joy change her own.

Joy encouraged me to call Dr. Bradley. I was skeptical but desperate. Joy explained to me that Dr. Bradley would help me. So, that night at about 10:00 p.m., I sent Dr. Bradley a long email requesting her help. I sent the email, not having any hope that she would be willing to help. The next morning when I awoke, I went to the computer filled with doubt that Dr. Bradley had even read my email, let alone replied. I could not believe my eyes when I saw the return email! She stated she would be glad to talk to me and show me the way!

I scheduled a phone conference with Dr. Bradley after filling out a health questionnaire. She shared her journey with me, her struggles with weight and food, and her mission to change one person at a time. Dr. Bradley encouraged me to take her *21-Day Vegan Challenge* program. I thought that if I could change myself, then I can change my family. It needed to start with me. Dr. Bradley assured me that I can do it, and I started her Challenge on May 2, 2015.

I shared with Dr. Bradley my frustration and that I didn't know where to begin or how to change my eating habits. I didn't know what I was doing wrong. I was already using some Vegan products. What I had not done was cut out the bad foods; meats, dairy, coffee, and sodas. *No coffee?* I was addicted to drinking that black cup of Joe! She advised me towards foods such as fruits and vegetables. She taught me to stay away from processed foods and outlined the healthy foods I was to consume. I also purchased her book *Kale Yeah It's Good*. I must tell you that I honestly felt like I was all thumbs and totally clueless about what to eat. With Dr. Bradley's one-on-one guidance, I slowly started understanding what foods to eat. Every day, I learned to make better choices.

After the 21 days, the best results came when my doctor noticed that all my numbers—like my blood pressure and A1C—went down. **Oh...and I started losing weight!** I had loads of energy and was finally feeling happy—*AND* my stomach was beginning to settle down.

Back to my daughter. Tara received a new kidney on May 4, 2017. She has stopped consuming processed foods, sodas, meats, and fast foods. My husband has also begun to eat healthier. His A1C has dropped back to normal and his doctor is lowering his daily medications. My husband is pleased with his diet change, all springing from the teachings and coaching I received from Dr. Bradley.

I started doing my own research to further my knowledge. I went on Netflix and found documentaries such as *Forks Over Knives* and *What the Health?* The documentaries helped me gain further knowledge and assurance that I was on the right track.

So, if you're thinking of changing your eating habits, *The 21-Day Vegan Challenge* is the way to go! Dr. Bradley has ignited in me a new passion for wanting to make healthy food choices and **not** follow the wrong ones.

I believe that a Vegan lifestyle is what man was chosen to eat from the beginning of time. Dr. Bradley has forever changed my life. I am excited and hope my testimony has encouraged, inspired, and motivated you to change. It is always a **"work in progress"**, but you're never too old to learn!

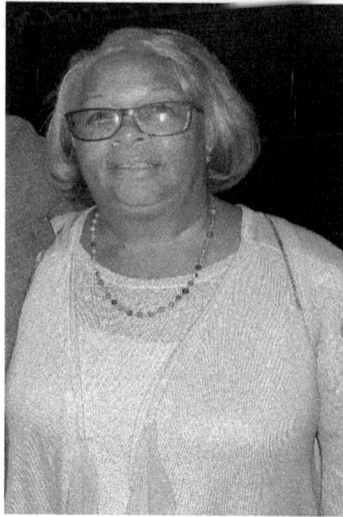

Ruth Tolbert grew up in Atlantic City, New Jersey. She is a former Dental Assistant and EMT/Paramedic. With a genuine love for helping people, she considers herself a Wellness Advocate and Humanitarian.

Ruth credits her grandmother for teaching her about holistic remedies for life's ailments. Carrying those teachings throughout her life, she seeks natural solutions — versus prescribing to pharmaceutical drugs that have harmful side-effects and would only 'manage' the symptoms; not cure them. She holds firmly to the belief that God has given us gifts from the earth and a host of natural foods and remedies on which to survive.

Contact Ruth Tolbert

Email: Belugafly1@aol.com

It's Not Over; The Journey Continues.
By Paulette Anderson

In October 2011, I made the decision to start making healthier lifestyle choices. I lost over 30 pounds and kept it off for almost a year. I found myself reaching a plateau, never really seeing any major transformation, even though I continued to go to the gym three to four days a week. I knew one of my issues even then was incorporating healthier food choices and monitoring what and when I ate. I've worked around wounded, ill, and injured soldiers for almost eight years, so I remembered being introduced to a Vegan lifestyle for the first time by a wounded soldier in 2012 who found it very difficult at that time to get a variety of healthy, plant-based food choices. He had to pay out-of-pocket and purchase things at a local Whole Foods store. He reached out to me for any veteran resources that could possibly help him with his out-of-pocket expenses.

In September 2015, Dr. Brenda—a dear high school classmate, sister, and friend—challenged some ladies to participate in a *21-Day Vegan Challenge* on Facebook beginning in October. I never thought it would be a turning point in my life's journey, but it was truly just what I needed **AND** at the right time (I had been diagnosed with Hyperthyroidism, a condition that caused severe bulging in both eyes which led to severe dry eyes. When she reached out to me, I was already preparing for eye surgery in both eyes to relieve some of the pressure.)

Committing to the Challenge, I initially felt afraid yet very hopeful about the positive results it would bring. Dr. Brenda promised us that she would be there every step of the way, and she did just that! With her help—constant encouragement, plant-based Trivia, and support videos and articles—I remained consistent for the **entire** 21 days. The key at the time was preparing my meals the night before, shopping for the week, and following most of the recipes and meal plans Dr. Brenda provided in her book. I was so full of energy, I continued with *another* 21 days in November, along with a seven-day cleanse that she invited us to participate in.

My first surgery on my right eye was in November on Veteran's Day, and my next surgery for the left eye was the week before Christmas. After both surgeries, the doctor stated he was truly amazed at how quickly I recovered with no complications nor concerns. I'm so thankful I accepted the Challenge. I truly believe it helped my body heal faster than it would have had I not prepared.

Two years later, I am now one of Dr. Brenda's original "Challengers". I can admit that I'm not consistent. I 'slip and fall' sometimes. I'm not yet fully committed to a plant-based lifestyle, but I continue to stay in the Helping Other People Evolve (H.O.P.E.) group page on Facebook. What I **can** tell you is this: Dr. Brenda and the H.O.P.E. group have been a blessing and have continued to provide me with tools, support, encouragement, and (most of all) **NO JUDGMENT!** So, I get back in the game and continue to incorporate healthy plant-based foods daily! I believe we must get the revelation in our own timing with God's help, while staying close to those who are consistent. It's a positive step in the right direction!

I wanted to share my 'gradual transformation' story with the hope that it may encourage someone in their journey to a healthier lifestyle. Today, I drink lots of lemon water, healthy smoothies, eat healthy snacks and meals, and exercise four to five days a week. For my 51st birthday, I signed up for and started attending an Over-40 Cross-Fit Group!

I thank God for His grace that sustains me through my continuous journey and for a life-partner of 31 years, Darrell, who supports, encourages, motivates, and keeps me going!

My favorite scripture during my journey is: *"Beloved, I PRAY that you may prosper in EVERY way and [that your body] may keep well, even as [I know] your SOUL keeps well and prospers!"* (3 John 1:2, AMP).

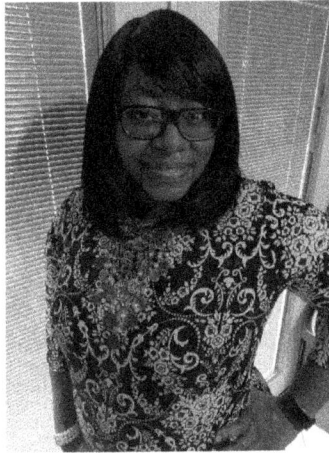

An Arkansas native who grew up singing in church, Paulette Anderson has had the privilege of singing encouraging songs to communities in the United States, Germany, France, Luxemburg, and Italy since 1988. In her music ministry, she has been a Choir Director, Lead Singer, and Praise and Worship Leader. She has led praise and worship during Women's Conferences in Oklahoma, Texas, and Washington, and had the honor of singing the National Anthem at several Lawton/Fort Sill events. She has been a guest speaker for a Woman's Retreat in Lawton, as well as during an all-night Prayer Meeting.

Paulette received her Bachelor's Degree in Theology from the Minnesota Graduate School of Theology through New Life Fellowship and attended the Ministry School in Oklahoma City under the International Pentecostal Holiness Church denomination.

Presently, Paulette works at Fort Sill's Reynolds Army Health Clinic as the MEDCOM Ombudsman, where she helps resolve any issues for soldiers and veterans in transition and their families. In her capacity, she serves as a neutral, independent, and impartial resource to them.

Paulette has been married to SFC Darrell T. Anderson, U.S. Army Retired, for over 31 years and has two children and two grandchildren.

She desires to see the Body of Christ celebrating 'Unity in Diversity' by doing all that God has called each of us to do! One of her favorite passages of Scripture is Ephesians 4:16 (NKJV, *Emphasis Added*):

*"…from whom the **WHOLE** body, joined and knit together by what **EVERY** joint supplies, according to the effective working by which every part does its share, causes **GROWTH** of the body for the edifying of itself in **LOVE**."*

Contact Paulette Anderson

Email: pauletteanderson66@gmail.com

My Yellow Brick Road to a Healthy Lifestyle
By Deborah Hassell

As a child, I thought *The Wizard of Oz* was a scary movie with ugly witches and monster monkeys. I was too young and inexperienced to understand the real message of the story: *All you need is within you – if you believe.* Dorothy and her friends always had what they needed within themselves: intelligence, a loving heart, and courage. Along their journey, wise people were there to help guide them on their way. As for me, I, too, have the intelligence, loving heart, and courage. I also had guides and experiences that assisted me all along the way.

The first guide was my grandfather who was born in the 1800s on Saba, a small Caribbean volcanic island. His people lived off the land by growing their food, using plants for medicine, and building their very lives with their bare hands. While in my teens, I remember occasions when my grandfather gave me natural medicine remedies for minor ailments. On one memorable occasion, I had eaten too much birthday cake. He advised me to drink fresh lemon water to stop the stomachache. The remedy worked! That was my awakening. I began to understand the **real** power of food.

I grew up during the 1960s—the beginning of the natural, vegetarian consciousness in urban America. Living in New York, there was a tremendous amount of information circulating and plenty of vegetarian restaurants offering foods made from scratch with fresh ingredients. I stopped eating red meat, pork, chicken, and fish in 1978.

My second guide was my daughter. She was born in 1978 and I knew I wanted to feed her good, nutritious baby food. Her birth motivated me to learn how to make and jar her baby food. I blended fresh vegetables and jarred all her baby food. During one of the visits to her pediatrician, after he had taken blood for a routine exam, he said, *"I don't know what you're doing, but keep it up!"* My baby was healthy. I did not feed her sugary snacks or cow's milk. She drank soy milk as an infant and toddler.

Funny sidebar about my family: They thought I was cruel because I didn't give her candy. Although I couldn't hold back outside influences, my daughter was a vegetarian until she was about three years old; however, the foundation of healthy eating was being laid.

In 1988, I moved to Dayton, Ohio—the Midwest...meat country! If it oinked, clucked, mooed, quacked, blew bubbles in the water—if it had parents, it was on the plate! And there is a fried recipe for almost **everything** you can cook. Even though I didn't go back to eating meat, I began to take shortcuts with processed prepared foods and eating out more often. I added fried fish back into my diet just because it was an easy carryout alternative to cooking. Plus, I love fried fish!

In 1990, I took a Cultural Leadership course offered by the City of Dayton. This course was my third guide. The intent of the course was to educate Dayton citizens on the diversity of the population. Each person had to write a research paper about a particular culture. I chose vegetarianism. My paper covered the different types of vegetarianism, the cultural influence on vegetarianism, and America's modern food-processing industry. That research sealed the deal! I could never eat meat again! My research revealed that most of what ends up on America's dinner table comes from modern industrial farms that housed **thousands** of chickens, pigs, cows, and other animals — disgusting places ran by companies whose only concern was their profit.

For the past seven years, I have been living with my life partner, David, who is a wonderful, loving man…and a major carnivore. He eats very few veggies; meats, beans, cheese, and condiments dominate his diet, topped off with an active sweet tooth. So, although I still don't eat meat, I began eating more dessert, pizza, and fast food. I was still a little overweight and feeling guilty about not being as conscientious as I knew I should be, but too lazy to make changes. I'm now in my mid-60s and very conscious that how I treat my body is now more important than ever. When we are younger, our bodies can compensate for our negligence, but that compensation decreases with age. I'm acutely aware of that fact.

When my fourth guide, Dr. Brenda's *21-Day Vegan Challenge*, presented itself in November 2016, I knew the Challenge would help me make the necessary changes to get back on track. In my circle of friends and acquaintances, there is only **one** other vegetarian (we don't see or talk to each other often). So, being connected to a community of people who had the same goals and shared their challenges and frustrations was a wonderful gift!

Once I committed to the Challenge, the first thing I had to do was an inventory of the food I had in the house. I know that eating well begins with the food you bring into the home. Surprisingly, I didn't have a lot of "bad" food, which really helped me see that my issue was with some of the frozen, pre-cooked supermarket foods and restaurant take-out food. I then chose a few recipes from Dr. Brenda's *Kale Yeah* cookbook.

The first challenge I faced was stocking my kitchen with Vegan foods and new spices. Some of those items were: Vegan cheeses, Vegan mayo, jackfruit, liquid amino, and extra-firm tofu. Veggie meat alternatives were already incorporated into my diet. I also included more organic foods (which are *very* expensive), but since I was shopping for myself, it wasn't too bad.

Shopping was interesting because I was not aware the major supermarkets had increased the shelf space for vegetarian foods. I found that health food stores are a good source for the spices because they sell them by the ounce, which is cheaper than the supermarkets. Health food stores also offer healthy convenience items such as pure (not from concentrate) lemon and ginger juices. I bought lots of fresh vegetables, but soon realized I had to change the **way** I shopped. Oftentimes, the vegetables would go bad because I didn't cook them soon after buying them (or because I was the only one eating them). If there were leftovers, they would go bad from not being consumed in a "timely" manner. Now, I buy small portions of vegetables and may have to visit the store a couple of times a week.

When I couldn't find canned jackfruit in Dayton, I bought a prepared seasoned jackfruit. I've tried two different flavors and didn't like either one. I love chickpeas, so the first recipe I tried was the "Not From the Sea Tuna". **I LOVE IT!** I've shared it with friends and they also love it. I've also made the Vegan cornbread and banana bread. Both were **great**!

Interesting note: I did not tell David the breads were Vegan. He didn't like the cornbread because he prefers more of a "cake-like" texture, but he **loved** the banana bread.

Now, let's talk 'cheese'. I love cheese, and Vegan cheese has been the biggest hurdle for me. Initially, I tried the Daiya non-dairy shredded and sliced cheese. It tasted like plastic to me. I then tried Go Veggie cheese, which is not Vegan because it contains milk protein. I liked that taste better than Daiya. Dr. Brenda recommended Daiya block cheddar, which isn't bad at all (I now buy the block cheddar and the cheddar slices). I've read that Go Veggie is now selling a Vegan cheese. I'll give that a try. What I learned many years ago is that some foods are an *acquired* taste — and that's not a bad thing.

What I love about completing the Challenge is that it has made me more adventurous with the foods I cook. I go online to find other Vegan recipes that include foods I've never cooked before like Yuca (or cassava), which my grandfather used to cook. Also, I planted a garden this Summer (raised planters I bought from Sam's Club) and grew collard greens, tomatoes, peppers, Swiss chard, and some herbs. It was a very good feeling picking fresh vegetables for my meals.

Thanks to Dr. Brenda, I am now building an inventory of essential oils to use medicinally and for aromatherapy. This has led to making my own lotions, deodorant, and lip balm. As I am more focused on being healthy, I have also been more conscientious about exercising. I am excited!

That is why my title is *"Yellow Brick Road"*. It is the path that **God** has for me. Trusting the guides and knowledge I encounter on my journey provides what I need for personal growth. Thank you, Dr. Brenda Bradley, for being my 'Glenda' (the Good Witch) and laying some of the most *beautiful* yellow bricks on my *"Yellow Brick Road"* journey!

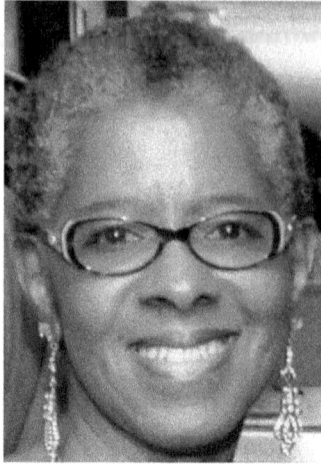

Deborah Hassell is a native New Yorker living joyously as a retiree in Dayton, Ohio. She loves to design jewelry, as well as instruct Detroit-style Urban Ballroom Dancing—an activity that allows her to add joy to the lives of others. Both activities nurture her creative spirit.

Deborah's vegetarian "Yellow Brick Road" journey began 40 years ago in her hometown of Bronx, New York. She states: "The 21-Day Vegan Challenge expanded my vegetarian lifestyle and opened a new door of creativity through the trying of new foods, making my own lotions, and learning about the benefits of essential oils."

Contact Deborah Hassell

Email: myopenheart@outlook.com

I Didn't Do This to Become a Vegan!
By Norman Ray

My life has been a true journey and full of things that have propelled me to be the best I could be! I've made so many changes in my life through the years, I can't begin to count. Early 2016, I had a health challenge that tried to suck the wind out of me, but I refused to allow myself to succumb to what was being related to me without **AT LEAST** meeting the battle head-on.

I had started a new project that I truly felt very good about. It ran along the line of women's health and a new product that was going to be introduced to North America that would literally have the ability to change many women's lives forever. It was during this period that I felt a strong desire to not only continue trying to be fit by going to the gym, but also find other ways to cut down on different types of food.

See, I was at a crossroad. How would I start a journey to live a healthier lifestyle without giving up some of the dishes I so enjoyed? It all started to come together one day when my wife and I were having dinner with a couple of friends from the great city of Philadelphia. During our conversation, we began to talk about eating habits and why it would be imperative to make lifestyle changes. We discussed things like eating more vegetables, fruits, nuts, and whole grains, while eliminating things such as meats, dairy products, and refined sugars. I truly walked away from that fellowship with a different perspective and life-altering thoughts.

In addition, while we were chatting about multiple issues associated with different foods and diets, my Sister-in-Christ, Mrs. Tolbert, mentioned an incredible lady that she fell in love with as a person and coach. She told me how since she had connected with her Doctor/Friend, her eating healthier was a life-saver — not only for her, but her family as well.

Ever since meeting 'this Doctor', I now have my own testimony on how talking to and connecting with her has changed my outlook on eating, dieting, and exercise. I've even begun to speak with others on the importance of healthy eating versus working out.

It wasn't until I was invited to partake in Dr. Brenda Bradley's *21-Day Vegan Challenge* that I truly began to see the need to work on me. During the time leading up to the Challenge, I was a man who worked out but still had eating habits that were counterproductive to all the hard work I was putting in. Also, during this time, I was experiencing a few "men challenges" that needed to be addressed. Unbeknownst to me, the challenges were (in many ways) linked to the foods I had been consuming...and *NOT* consuming. What really shocked me was that I found many of my issues — and other folks' issues, too — were related to the meats we love to eat!

So, after I discovered my dysfunction, I went to work. I partook of *The 21-Day Vegan Challenge* and, in doing so, began to see results like no other. My male "drive" began to be rekindled and, of course, the belly began to decrease to the point where I could look down and see my belt buckle! It may sound funny, but just think: If you can't see your belt buckle, just imagine what else could be hindered with a slightly round stomach!

While on the Challenge, I began to experiment in the kitchen and created some truly wonderful different types of salads, along with meals that not only did I enjoy, but my wife as well! What's even better is that through this journey, others who are connected to me on social media were inspired and began to take the journey with us! This was truly amazing and life-changing!

Now, I must admit that since *The 21-Day Vegan Challenge*, I've consumed red meat. I ate it once and it didn't sit right with my "new-and-improved digestive system", so **THAT** is gone! As it relates to consuming other meats, it's minimum (if at all). I no longer touch processed meats and have not had breakfast meats since *The 21-Day Vegan Challenge*—not even turkey products. For me, this is amazing! I must be truthful and say I still eat a little fish and dairy, but only about once or twice a week (if that).

My "sorry" is that I didn't do this to become a Vegan; it was to see if I could change a habit and get on a healthier regimen. In my mind and heart, I've achieved my goal and will continue to strive for greater.

So, for all you folks who either know me (and for those who don't), my journey is not over. A new way of putting foods into my body has forever changed the way I consume and think about food. What I've also learned is that even when I slip, I will not condemn myself. It's like the Word tells us in Romans 8:1 (KJV), *"Therefore, there is now no condemnation for those who are in Christ Jesus"*—meaning don't allow yourself nor anyone else to condemn or keep you in a state of conviction. Brush yourself off and keep moving towards your success.

Lastly, I want to thank God, my wife and children, and my coach, Dr. Bradley. Without all of you, this would have been a much more difficult challenge. I must not forget Mrs. Ruth Tolbert. If it were not for her, I wouldn't have even thought about a way to change my eating habits and the associated pleasure of being connected to Dr. Brenda Bradley.

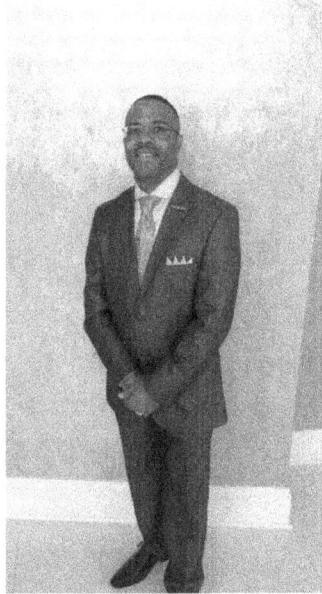

Norman J. Ray was born and raised in Baltimore, Maryland. He joined the United States Army in 1978, where he held an illustrious career of 22 years working in various fields to include Signal Corp, Food Service, and Training Developer Writer. He is presently employed with the Defense Logistics Agency in Richmond, Virginia.

Norman holds a Bachelor's Degree in Individualized Studies from Virginia State University; an Applied Science Degree in Food Service Management from Central Texas College; and is a graduate of Ever-Increasing Training Center with a Diploma in Biblical Studies. He also serves as a Minister at Mt. Gilead Full Gospel International Ministries under the covering of Bishop Daniel Robertson, Jr. and Co-Pastor Elena Robertson in Richmond, Virginia where they are changing lives with the Word of God.

Norman is 38 years married (and counting) to the beautiful Denise A. Ray. They have two adult children; Anthony and Amaya Ray, and a daughter-in-law; Nikkia Ray. He is the proud grandfather of two grandchildren: Jiselle and Jason Ray.

Contact Norman J. Ray

Email: normanray@verizon.net

Twitter: @NormanRay3

Sick and Tired of Being Sick and Tired!
By Kenya M. Sumner

I was never a heavyset person. I certainly did not want to become one. My mother has been plus-sized most of my life, and I didn't want that for myself. At the onset of weight gain, I would do what I thought I needed to do to prevent it. That meant cutting certain foods out of my diet, finding a quick weight-loss scheme, and exercising. Those were *temporary* solutions. I needed **long-term** changes.

I started on my road to weight loss and healthier living in September 2014. I noticed I had gained some weight, and my body began to hurt as a result. The sides of my body along my midsection and my back were in constant pain. I had never felt pain like that before, nor had I ever experienced pains in those areas of my body. It was new and I **hated** it! I would look at myself in the mirror and didn't like what I saw looking back at me. I was changing…and not for the better. I also found myself being tired a lot. Getting up to start the day was a bigger challenge than usual, and starting *any* project was like pushing a heavy boulder over a hill to get to the other side, when all I had to do was walk around it.

I enjoyed coffee and the effects of caffeine, so I attempted to overcome the low energy by consuming more than my usual one small cup of coffee per day. Before I knew it, I was ordering multiple cups throughout the day. My caffeine consumption had gotten so bad that one day, a large intake of caffeine led to a full-on anxiety attack, complete with uncontrolled body shaking.

I had had enough. That day, I asked my sorority sister for help. She had just begun her own journey to becoming a Lifestyle/Fitness Coach, and her timing couldn't have been any better! She got me started on the program she was advising her clients to go through. Like so many good starts, I did not continue with her program. By January of the following year, I was back to my old eating habits. I did manage to continue exercising, with a preference for running. While running gave me energy, it wasn't enough. I soon stopped that, too, and never quite returned to being consistent with my exercise plan.

Over the course of 2015 and 2016, I tried the Daniel Fast, juicing fasts, the lemonade diet, the vegetarian diet, and being a Vegan—when it was *convenient* for me. I still kept some type of exercise plan in place, but again: I wasn't consistent enough to see long-lasting results.

In September 2017, I had another moment of desperation. Compensating (again) for a lack of energy, this time choosing that "high energy drink" (R*d B**l) to be my 'medicine', I again overindulged and had another anxiety attack. This time, I looked at my life in its totality. I was consuming more alcohol than usual, drinking energy drinks, feeling depressed, gaining weight, and I had stopped running altogether. Once again, I needed help.

I had just seen Dr. Brenda at a mutual friend's house party. I had known Brenda for a few years, and she had been a Vegan ever since I met her. Every time we saw each other, we talked about her lifestyle. I wanted so much to be a part of that life, but I wasn't ready at the time. In September 2017, I was ready.

I called Dr. Brenda because she mentioned to me that she had a *21-Day Vegan Challenge* program. I was at my wits end and was sick and tired of being sick and tired. I wanted to give her program a try. I was both excited and nervous because I had *tried* to be a Vegan before. I *tried* to cut out the dairy and meat...I *tried* to leave the cheese alone! Well, I now realize those weren't attempts to change my lifestyle; they were changes in my meal choices—for that day. I knew I had to be consistent and go through a **real** change.

I made sure I could financially complete the Challenge and mentally face any hurdles that may come my way. I didn't know what I was in for, but I tried my best to prepare for anything.

The 21-Day Vegan Challenge was the transformation I needed! Dr. Brenda would tell me she couldn't wait for me to see my true self. In the beginning, I didn't know what she was talking about. After taking the Challenge, I "see" myself. I "see" a beautiful woman. I "see" a beautiful body. I "see" that I can live off of the goodness that has already been prepared by God for us! They are found in nature! I love my new life as a Vegan!

The immediate changes I saw were the lifting of what I call the "morning fog". Before I became a Vegan, I was so tired in the morning, I could not part my mouth to speak! I would put up a two-finger peace sign when it was my turn to respond to a *"Good Morning!"* It would take me **at least** 30 minutes to wake up after the last alarm went off. I would lay in bed, motionless and stiff, until the "fog" lifted. Thank goodness: That is no longer a part of my life! I enjoy the blessing and possibility of what the morning brings. I am forever grateful.

I do not take this lifestyle lightly. I am more consistent in the things I pursue and, more importantly, the things I put in my body. I don't worry about being a heavyset person because my lifestyle doesn't lend itself to being plus-sized. I still have my flaws, but those flaws don't keep me static; they keep me in check as I travel the road to optimal health!

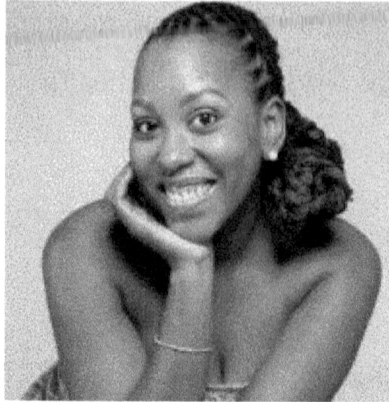

"I love TV!" is a common quote of Mrs. Kenya M. Sumner, so she decided to join the ranks of those brave souls behind the lens.

One of Kenya's first jobs out of college was at CBS, where she was a Legal Assistant. She assisted the legal staff on King World, producing shows like *Inside Edition, The Ananda Lewis Show,* and *Curtis Court.*

Kenya then moved to Maryland and briefly attended the Corcoran College of Art and Design, majoring in Graphic Design. It was there that she honed in on her creative eye and developed new ways to "think outside the box". While in Maryland, she was blessed to become an entrepreneur and opened 'Prep for Filming', a production rental equipment company. Upon her return to her first joy, television production, she has worked on television commercials including those for Nike, United Way, and the 2006 Super Bowl Halftime Show.

Kenya is a graduate of Howard University in Washington, D.C., and is a self-employed Production Manager. She has worked on the BET Honors, Soul Train Awards, and in performance at White House concerts.

Kenya currently resides in Clinton, Maryland with her husband and daughter.

Contact Kenya M. Sumner

Email: kenyamarie.farmer@gmail.com

Facebook: www.facebook.com/kenyamarie.farmer

Instagram: @prepforfilming

Twitter: @prepforfilming

THIS PAGE INTENTIONALLY LEFT BLANK

My Journey to Fabulous Fifty Starts NOW!
By Tamara McCutcheon

"T*he Slaves got their allowance every Monday night of molasses, meat, corn, meal, and a kind of flour called 'dredgings' or 'shorts'. Perhaps this allowance would be gone before the next Monday night, in which case the slaves would steal hogs and chickens. Then would come the whipping-post. Master himself never whipped his slaves; this was left to the overseer. We children had no supper, and only a little piece of bread or something of the kind in the morning. Our dishes consisted of one wooden bowl, and oyster shells were our spoons. This bowl served for about fifteen children, and often the dogs and the ducks and the peafowl had a dip in it. Sometimes we had buttermilk and bread in our bowl, sometimes greens or bones*" (Burton, 1909).

Those are the words of Annie L. Burton, a slave girl recounting her happy life in her chapter, *Memories of Childhood's Slavery Days*, in the book *Women's Slave Narratives*. One hundred eight years later, I write as a woman who grew up in the south, just as young Annie did. Generations of African-Americans, including my beloved family, adopted the slavery-influenced diets of eating flesh (pork, beef, and chicken) and the by-product of flesh such as eggs, cheese, and milk. As a community, we've continued eating a diet that has and continues to kill us. African-Americans are the group most affected by obesity, heart disease, cancer, diabetes, and hypertension—conditions I grew up thinking was a *'Black Thing'* when, in essence, it's a **'Diet Thing'**. Wisdom comes with age, and as I embark on a half century of life, I've finally decided to take control of my nutrition and pursue a plant-based diet!

My name is Tamara McCutcheon. I am a proud Air Force retiree. I served our nation for 26 years. As Maya Angelou so eloquently stated, *"I am the HOPE and the DREAM of the slave"*. I've made it a lifelong obligation to excel at every endeavor I face in an effort to uplift my community. I stand on the shoulders of the ancestors…I stand on the shoulders of that little girl, Annie L. Burton, who couldn't fathom what a young black girl would accomplish in America this present day. However, the remnants of slavery are still present in my life when I sit at the dinner table.

I grew up in South Carolina—60 miles south of 'ChuckTown'. Charleston, South Carolina is where 40-60% of the Africans landed when they were brought to America. There's no secret to why my family continues to consume a harmful diet: We like to **EAT**! My grandfather fed his family raising hogs. I helped slaughter a baby hog as a child (I'm still traumatized), and enjoyed pit barbeque…until it made me sick. It made a lot of us sick, even though we were warned to not eat too much of it. The warning should have been to not eat it **at all**. Don't get me wrong: Cooking with salt pork and throwing a hamhock in your collard greens or cabbage is quite tasty — and there's nothing I wouldn't do to have a plate of my mother's food right now if I could. She was the *ultimate* cook…the one person everyone lauded. Her dishes were the ones you looked for on Thanksgiving. Her cakes (cooked with eggs from chickens raised on our farm) were the closest thing to Heaven you could get on earth. The tagline 'Melt in Your Mouth' was meant for her delectable chocolate cake; **not** M&M candies. As pleasing to the palette as her cooking may have been, it definitely wasn't conducive to healthy nutrition.

When I left South Carolina at the young age of 18 for the Air Force, I always looked for the Soul Food spots. I wanted a taste of home: ***food smothered in fat.*** Although I dealt with chronic stomach pain my entire life, I still continued eating unhealthy foods. At least once every several months, I found myself eating soup and crackers because my stomach was revolting against me. I couldn't hold food down and dealt with constant bouts of diarrhea and pain. I've had several colonoscopies, fearful I had cancer. Thankfully, I've always come up clear.

My body was constantly combating what I was feeding it. I absolutely loved steak. I was an epicurean when it came to fine cuts of beef. I sought out the finest steak houses wherever I found myself stationed. Halls Chophouse in Charleston, South Carolina; Charlie Palmers in Washington, D.C.; and Coach & Four in Ft. Walton Beach, Florida were my favorite dining spots…just to name a few. I would eat some form of beef several times a week, all the while dealing with stomach pain because I thought I had a 'weak stomach' since I'd been that way since childhood. At the time of this writing, it's been over a year since I've had beef.

Another health issue I dealt with—one I feel is **directly** tied to diet—is fibroids. I was first told I had fibroids during an annual exam/pap smear. The male doctor said it was no big deal and not to worry until I was ready to have children. I did some preliminary research and, since I didn't have any symptoms at the time, I didn't worry about it. A year later, my symptoms were prominent. I had such an extreme case of fibroids, at the age of 31, I found myself in the hospital on the verge of getting a blood transfusion. I was severely anemic, barely walking around with a blood level count of 4.5 (it should have been 12.5). My weight had dropped to 140 pounds (I looked like a skeleton), I was bleeding for 30 days straight, I had absolutely no appetite, and I found myself having dizzy spells several times a day. I finally got an **excellent** doctor who said, *"Let's see why you're losing blood"*. I refused the transfusion until further investigation. She immediately placed me on iron pills, and my blood count went up. She determined the issue was fibroids.

As a whole, the medical community still doesn't know what exactly causes fibroids. Experts agree fibroids develop and are caused by impure blood, unbalanced diet, and constipation. Fibroids grow on diets based on the consumption of meat and dairy. African-American women have the highest occurrence of fibroids compared to other groups.

As I was diagnosed and treated, the discussion of changing my diet **NEVER** came up. I never took a moment to connect the dots myself. The first operation I underwent was Uterine Fibroid Embolization. Six years later, the fibroids were back with a vengeance. At the age of 39, I had a Laparoscopic Hysterectomy.

After a lifetime battling stomach issues, in 2014, I was finally diagnosed with Irritable Bowel Syndrome. The doctor giving the diagnosis **STILL** didn't feel compelled to discuss changing my diet. He suggested taking probiotics to balance the good versus the bad bacteria in my intestinal tract — but (as stated in my opening paragraph)…with age comes wisdom. I had already begun taking steps toward eating healthier, starting with the elimination of beef from my diet a year prior. I've known for quite some time that returning to the diet Annie and my ancestors followed *before* landing in Charleston, South Carolina is paramount. The ancestors lived and thrived on a plant-based lifestyle, from diet to medicines.

In July 2017, I took Dr. Bradley's *21-Day Vegan Challenge*. My body was elated! I immediately lost 20 pounds, which was severely needed because for the first time in my life, I was tipping the scales at over 200 pounds. My 'Love Handles' aren't as loveable now. My skin is much clearer. I don't feel as sluggish because I sleep better. The immediate, positive effects of miniscule changes to healthy eating cannot be denied. I still eat a piece of salmon or grilled chicken on my salad a couple times a week. I've given myself six months (or less) to totally eliminate meat. I have to set realistic goals for myself so I'm not beating myself up each time I bite into a piece of chicken. I know I'll get there!

I have to work on the discipline of preparation, cooking, and going to the grocery store. Singlehood has made me a slave to convenience. However, as the title of my chapter emphatically states: **My Journey to Fabulous Fifty Starts NOW!** My health is my greatest wealth. The transition to a plant-based diet has already manifested great results, and I'm not turning back.

Why would I? **I FEEL GOOD!**

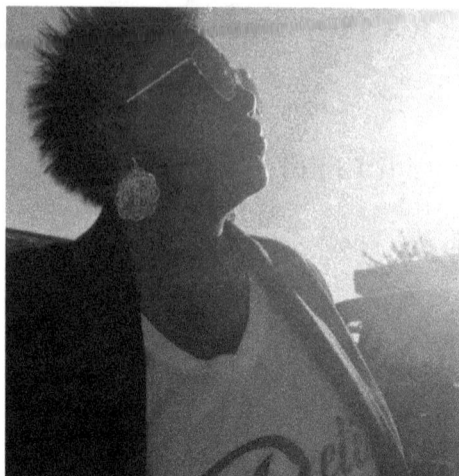

Tamara McCutcheon retired from the United States Air Force on January 1, 2014 after a rewarding 26-year career. She progressed quickly through the ranks and held a myriad of leadership positions. Her last job was Flight Commander, Plans & Integration, 53rd Computer Systems Squadron at Eglin AFB, Florida.

After retirement, Tamara relocated to Charleston, South Carolina. There, she continued to serve others as a community volunteer. She was a pivotal member of the SC Governor's special cadre of Guardian ad Litems (GaL); child advocates for children in the Department of Social Services system. As a GaL, Tamara played a vital role in a Governor-sponsored initiative to become a voice for children at risk. She also volunteered with the YWCA Street Outreach program in downtown Charleston. Her efforts were paramount in forging the fight to eradicate homelessness in Charleston, South Carolina. She worked closely with many homeless veterans to get their lives back on track.

Tamara envisioned RETIRED CHICKs, LLC (RC) immediately after retirement, but 'life happened'. Overcoming personal challenges and setbacks, she decided to relocate to Hampton, Virginia in May 2017. In June 2017, she initiated a business page on Facebook and launched her entrepreneurship journey. The mission of RETIRED CHICKs, LLC is to 'Inspire & Empower' Women Worldwide. Proceeds will benefit organizations and charities that are championing causes for women and children (from homelessness to mentorship programs and everything in between). RETIRED CHICKs, LLC is a creative mix of apparel/product sales, a social media platform, varied business ventures, and collaboration with other organizations to reach mission success.

Contact Tamara McCutcheon

Facebook: www.facebook.com/RETIREDCHICKs

THIS PAGE INTENTIONALLY LEFT BLANK

Testimony of a 21-Day Vegan Challenger
By Rosemary Hill

Blessed by Dr. Brenda T. Bradley's call to give a testimony of my journey during the October 2017 *21-Day Vegan Challenge*, my first thought was that it was a huge honor. Then, the following scripture came to mind: *"For unto whomever much is given, of him shall much be required"* (Luke 12:48, KJV). One word can possess great meaning and, when put with other words, can produce a powerful testimony.

The dictionary gives a few meanings of the word 'testimony':

1. Something that is written or spoken statement, especially one given in the court of law or evidence; or
2. Proof provided by the existence or appearance of something; or
3. A public recount of religious conversion or experience.

In all instances, a testimony is a very serious and impactful way of sharing a message or recalling an experience. My testimony to you is not one of a legal nature, nor is it a matter of spirituality. It is one I hope will be stimulating and impactful so much that you will take heed and want to experience it for yourself.

My *21-Day Vegan Challenge* journey began when I signed up for the November 2016 Challenge. I had friends who were Vegans and often when we went to lunch, I would try something plant-based. When I learned about the Challenge, I decided to sign up for my birthday. What better timing? I have found that oftentimes, I look for opportunities to make fresh starts, so the gift to myself at the age of 45 was learning to eat healthier.

Prior to signing up for the Challenge, my dynamics were that for years, I cooked what I thought were healthy meals for my family. The meals I prepared consisted of a meat of some sort, a starch, and a vegetable. For the kids, they had a glass of milk to help them grow big and strong. I grew up eating 'traditional' southern foods, so what I fed my family was a derivative of what I ate while growing up.

After serving 15 years in the United States Army, I thought myself to be fit and (more importantly) I thought I tweaked a few meals to make them healthier. Instead of frying foods, I baked and incorporated vegetables that I didn't even eat growing up. I considered myself one who made healthy meals for my family.

Going into the Challenge, I spoke with my children about what I was going to do and discussed with them what I knew about plant-based eating. The discussion prompted me to research the benefits in depth so that I would know for myself, but also to share with others who may want to know about the Challenge. I learned that eating plant-based foods was good for those who were obese, Type-2 diabetic, suffered from cardiovascular disease, and/or had high blood pressure.

To be honest, I had none of those conditions. I was 5'6" tall and weighed 140 pounds. My concern was more about how I would get the right protein and calorie intake so that I would **NOT** lose weight. There was so much for me to learn about replacing my foods and not giving them up.

As a 'Challenger', I was initially intimidated and even overwhelmed with shopping for the various foods that were in Dr. Bradley's cookbook. I did not know how to prepare the meals, but I slowly began to see the transition of foods in my cupboards and the refrigerator. I had to find a new grocery store to shop for foods because the place where I shopped did not have the types of foods I needed to eat (if they did, choices were very limited).

In all things, preparation is key. Meal preparation added to my success of the Challenge because there were many times when a "quick snack" could have easily meant going to the nearby vending machine or eating donuts or cake brought into the office by someone. I noticed that the meat took the longest to prepare, so I even saved **time** in the evening by making plant-based meals.

Things that helped me be successful in the Challenge included Dr. Bradley's *Kale Yeah* cookbook and the interactive group chat on Facebook. Dr. Bradley posted thought-provoking questions about various foods and caused us to question the foods we had been eating. She reminded us, *"Your food should be your medicine"*. By eating plant-based foods, they would provide all the vitamins and nutrients we needed.

The group members were encouraging to one another and Dr. Bradley was there to answer questions and keep us informed about what our bodies have been going through daily. She provided insight and encouragement daily, so we 'Challengers' were never without information.

I took the Challenge for the first time in November 2016. I continued to eat *somewhat* plant-based, but reverted to some foods that I missed so much. I found there was a difference in the way I felt and the clarity I had as it related to being creative and energetic, so I took *The 21-Day Vegan Challenge* **again** in October 2017. That time, it was to assist in my full transition into the Vegan lifestyle. I am happy to report that my weight loss was minimal, but only because I purposefully increased my calorie intake to maintain my weight.

I continue to participate in the group chats to encourage new Challengers while continuing to learn about plant-based eating. Overall, I feel empowered by the information learned. I feel inspired to pass along what I have learned to others and feel that now is my time to share my experience.

I am a *21-Day Vegan Challenger* **Finisher**. These words make up my testimony.

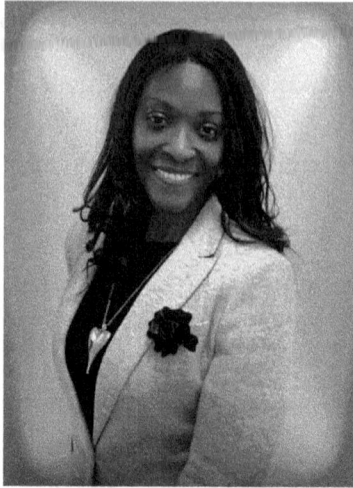

Rosemary Hill's career started when she joined the United States Army in 1989. Initially, she served three years as a Medical Supply Specialist, after which she was then trained as a Unit Supply Specialist. She deployed to Kuwait and served honorably until 2005 when she exited the military to become and Acquisition and Contracting Professional.

Rosemary is currently the Deputy Director of Contracting, supporting various Army programs. She manages day-to-day contracting operations and evaluates program effectiveness to identify potential areas of improvement to better meet the unique needs of the organization. She also provides expert acquisition and procurement advice and recommendations to the Director and other Senior Leaders within the organization on procurement and contract matters.

Rosemary holds a Level III certification in Contracting from the Defense Acquisition University, a B.A. in Acquisition in Contracting from Strayer University, and an M.A. in Acquisition and Contracting from Webster University. At the time of this writing, she is preparing to take the exam to become a Certified Federal Contracts Manager in the National Contract Management Association.

Rosemary is the mother of three children; Ashley (26), David, Jr. (24), and Amber (19). She takes pride in being a mother and enjoys writing, exercising, and has a passion for supporting her family, friends, and community.

Contact Rosemary Hill

Email: Legacibuilder@gmail.com

THIS PAGE INTENTIONALLY LEFT BLANK

The 40-Day Vegan
By Timothy Neal

For several years, I have been eating clean and trying different diets, waffling between Whole 30, Paleo, and *"I'll just have one carb serving today"*. I was successful in all of my diet endeavors, especially the Paleo diet. I meal-prepped daily (which is required for all healthy-eaters) and became a decent cook. Through all of the clean eating, I kept a steady workout regimen, combining Crossfit and Brazilian Jiu-Jitsu.

After clean-eating for a while, I began to notice that when I ate junk (pizza, chips, bread, and cookies), my belly would swell and I wouldn't perform well at the gym. I would have a sluggish feeling for hours, to the point that physical activity that day wouldn't happen.

When eating clean and working out, one begins to be in tune with their body. What I mean by that is this: When foreign food is consumed, you feel its effects immediately. You feel it hit your stomach and the effect it has on your blood sugar. My focus continued to be on my belly bloat. Even while eating Paleo, I would still get a belly bloat at times. I thought, *"There MUST be a better way!"* I wanted to try a different way of eating; a challenge. I decided to try *The 21-Day Vegan Challenge*.

Over several years, I have watched Dr. Bradley transform herself into a lean, strong, and healthy woman. I decided I wanted to give *The 21-Day Vegan Challenge* a try and reached out to her through Facebook. I signed up for her next Challenge.

My *21-Day Vegan Challenge* began on April 3rd and ended on May 13th. I felt so good, I decided to keep the Challenge going for **40 days**! For me, the most difficult days during the Challenge were days three and four. As my body began to detox, I was feeling nauseated and tired. Just think: Four days of **ZERO** animal by-product and your body gets angry? Still, I stayed the course and didn't give up. By day seven, I was great! My tummy was no longer swollen. Best of all, I could feel a difference in my legs — an unexpected benefit!

I describe myself as a meat-lover. I love all things bacon and chicken. If you add some bacon and butter to 'anything', it makes it that much better! I thought there was no way I could get through the Challenge... Prior to the Challenge, every weekday included something chicken, and every weekend, bacon. My daughter adopted my love for bacon as well. Even during the Challenge, I would cook some slices for her — but I never gave in to the temptation. Eventually, that temptation was gone. My cravings were replaced with fruit and oatmeal for breakfast. It only took 12 days to break the habit.

Gym days during those 40 days were **outstanding**! I didn't have to warm up. My legs didn't feel sluggish as they usually did the first 15 minutes on the mat. I could walk on the mat and just "GO"! Prior to the Challenge, my warm-ups included a lot of grunting and joint-popping before I began simple jumping jacks. Easy movements like jogging were met with challenges. The way I now feel can only be attributed to the Vegan way: Less meat in my diet meant less muscle tension and tightness.

The 21-Day Vegan Challenge diet consisted of a lot of leafy greens, sweet potatoes, and beans. My digestive system began to get clean and regular. Fruits and steel-cut oatmeal were great snacks as well. Learning what quick, on-the-go snacks were best when eating Vegan was fun. For me, almonds were always handy. I soon became an expert at reading food labels at the supermarket or looking for the "Vegan label" on packaging.

Fortunately, I had three weeks of travel to southern California, which I consider Vegan Wonderland. Every restaurant I visited had several Vegan options. I ate some of the best meals of the year while visiting. Usually, when traveling, it's more difficult to plan. Many times, I would eat dried fruit from service stations if I was on a road trip.

Eating clean is not easy. It takes a lot of meal planning, recipe planning, grocery shopping, cooking, and packing. It becomes a part-time job! Remember this: You have **ONE** body. Take care of it as if it were your newborn baby. You wouldn't feed your child poison, would you?

The 21-Day Vegan Challenge has taught me to make better food choices in my daily life. I challenge each of you reading this book to challenge yourself and go Vegan. You will have days when you give in to your old ways; just remember to stay on track and stick to your meal plan.

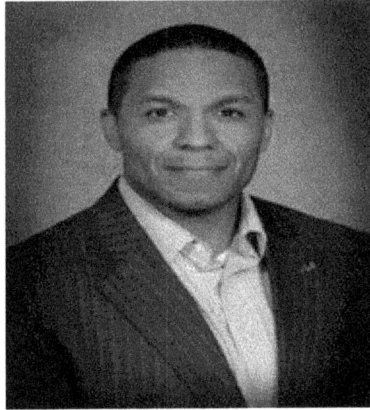

Originally from West Virginia, Timothy Neal has resided in the Washington, DC Metro area for 17 years. He holds a Bachelor of Science Degree in Management from Fairmont State University and currently works for a government contractor in the DC suburbs.

Timothy has one daughter, Natalie, who is a third-grader. He enjoys practicing Brazilian Jiu Jitsu and, as time permits, Crossfit.

Contact Timothy Neal

Instagram: @143nmit

CONCLUSION

As I write these final words, I have lived on this earth for 50 years. Recently, while thinking back over my life, I realized that I never fully understood how to care for my body. After leaving home, I still didn't know how to properly care for my body and, over the course of time, began to watch it deteriorate. I suffered from many ailments and recall getting sick over and over again.

One day, during an appointment, I recall my doctor telling me that I was borderline diabetic, had high blood pressure, high cholesterol, and was weighing 236 pounds. She advised me to lose weight, but couldn't instruct me on **HOW** to lose the weight. This was very puzzling because I had tried many things and couldn't lose the weight and keep it off. I was embarrassed and ashamed. I knew that it was only a matter of time before depression came knocking.

There were many days and nights I questioned God and felt that He stopped hearing my prayers. I started feeling sorry for myself, combined with all the physical, mental, and emotional abuse I had experienced during the last 44 years of my life. Although I felt as if God no longer heard my cries, I never stopped praying. I asked God to *please* show me what to do—and I promised to do it. Not too much longer after that, I was introduced to a plant-based lifestyle and haven't looked back since.

Being sick and overweight caused low self-esteem, depression, and diminished my quality of life. Many people are sick and dying. Food has the amazing power to both create and destroy health. We put all manner of animal products into our bodies, which are loaded with fat containing all the toxins from everything that animal has eaten during its entire lifetime—not to mention the antibiotics and growth hormones that were introduced into that animal's body. The animal fat within these products accumulate in our bodies, clog our arteries, and cause death due to heart attacks, strokes, etc.

It's been several years since I stopped eating meat. I **never** thought I could give up meat, fish, eggs, milk, and cheese; but after losing 33 pounds during the first 40 days, I am convinced this journey will last a lifetime. I am not an expert, but I am willing to help others who are willing to commit and understand this is not an easy journey—and that the rewards are great!

~ Dr. Brenda T. Bradley ~

APPENDIX

Angelou, M. (1978). *Still I Rise*. Random House Publishing, Manhattan, New York.

Burton, A.L. (1909). *Women's Slave Narratives*. Memories of Childhood's Slavery Days, pp. 4. Dover Publishing, Mineola, New York.

Testimony. (n.d.). Retrieved November 19, 2017, from https://www.merriam-webster.com/dictionary/testimony

www.ingramcontent.com/pod-product-compliance
Lightning Source LLC
Chambersburg PA
CBHW071239020426
42333CB00015B/1544